FRAGRANCES OF THE SOUL

The Attari Tradition of Therapeutic Perfume

John E Smith

Strategic Book Publishing and Rights Co.

Strategic Book Publishing and Rights Co., LLC
USA | Singapore
www.sbpra.net

For information about special discounts for bulk purchases, please contact Strategic Book Publishing and Rights Co. Special Sales, at bookorder@sbpra.net.

ISBN: 978-1-68235-283-0

Book Design: Suzanne Kelly

CONTENTS

FOREWORD V

INTRODUCTION vii

CHAPTER ONE 1
So Where Do I Start?

CHAPTER TWO 5
The Origins of Therapeutic Perfume

CHAPTER THREE 11
*Natural Perfumes Used in the Healing Traditions
of India, China, and Japan*

CHAPTER FOUR..18
Herbal Medicine, as Old as the Ark

CHAPTER FIVE 26
The Persian Tradition

CHAPTER SIX..31
Attars of Arabia

CHAPTER SEVEN 35
Sacred Scents

CHAPTER EIGHT 44
Fragrances of the Season—The Florals

CHAPTER NINE..50
Base Notes—Woody and Resinous Attars

CHAPTER TEN..53
Fragrance in the Time of COVID-19

CHAPTER ELEVEN
The Exotics...57

John E Smith

CHAPTER TWELVE 62
    Pure Perfume (Attars) to Enhance Presence,
    Confidence, and Well-Being

REFERENCES 66

END NOTES 68

FOREWORD

Isis, Lotus, Saraswathi.
Tree musk, amber, agarbathi.
Brother Thyme and Sister Cistus.
Myrrh of Mary, Gold of Christus.

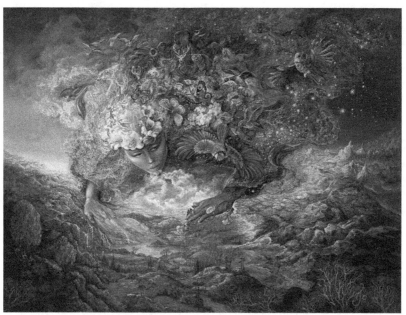

"Breath of Gaia" (c) Josehine Wall

In the beginning She created perfume, from the fragrance of the fig, the resins of Juniper, the lichens, the mosses and the earth itself after the rains. And She smelled that it was good.

The angels of the air, the earth, the fire and the water, brought to her their treasures. The angels of the air brought breath, "Ruh," spirit. The angel of the earth carried gemstones, spikenard and khus. The angel of fire brought her alembics, her crucibles. And the angel of water brought her pearls, coral and ambergris.

"In extracting the oils, the angels take their share." [1]

INTRODUCTION

Some years ago, I became aware that there was not a comprehensive book available on the Attari tradition (at least not in English). I had been working with attars in my herbal practice for some years, so I decided to write such a book.

My earlier books, *100 Herbs of Power* and *Food, Herbs, Health and Healing*, both included a small section on the therapeutic use of attars, but these merely introduced the subject.

After giving a lecture on Unani Tibb (Middle Eastern medicine) and Avicenna's use of perfume attars, one of my students asked me to recommend a book on the subject. I told him that there was no such thing (my apologies to Mandy Aftel, Lise Manniche, Julia Lawless, Jennifer Peace Rhind, Peter Holmes, and other authoritative writers and scholars whose work I hadn't read at that stage—an oversight since remedied). Anyway, this is for you, Tom, for encouraging me to write this text (albeit ten years later), and for you, Jay (who went as far as setting me a timeline).

CHAPTER ONE

So Where Do I Start?

My first experience of pure attars was in Pakistan in 1972, a time of great upheaval due to the Bangladesh war.

I had boarded a train at a rural station. A man who boarded later started a long conversation that we continued for a couple of hours. When he left the train at another rural station, he said he would like to give me a gift and handed me a tiny vial of a most exquisite perfume attar, which I carried with me for many months, enjoying its fragrance, until it finally disappeared (I think it was during a police search in the Belgrade railway station).

Around twenty years later, I made a study of attars with a hakim from the Unani Tibb tradition. When I completed my study, the hakim sent me a gift—the very same fragrance I had received in Pakistan. I still have some.

"There are scents that linger for decades—a cupboard rubbed with musk, a piece of leather drenched with cinnamon oil, a blob of ambergris, a cedar chest— they will possess virtually eternal olfactory life. While other things—lime oil, bergamot, jonquil and tuberose extracts, and many floral scents—evaporate within a few hours if they are exposed to the air in a pure, unbound form. The perfumer counteracts this fatal circumstance by binding scents that are too volatile by putting them in chains, so to speak, taming their urge for freedom— though this art consists of leaving enough slack in the chains for the odour simply to preserve its freedom even when it is tied so deftly that it cannot flee." [2]

One of my earliest attars was a tree musk bought in Varanasi in the early 1970s. I found a small amount of this in the back of a cupboard thirty or forty years later; it still smelled as strong, if not stronger, as when I bought it.

After three thousand years in King Tut's tomb, the unguent jars were opened—they were still fragrant.

* * *

Attar is an Arabic word meaning fragrance or essence. Attars are traditionally prepared by cold rolling in stone troughs (the plant materials used are replaced several times during the process to create a high concentration of their essences) or by steam distillation in degs (traditional stills with copper lids sealed with cotton and clay); both of these methods have been used for nearly a thousand years.

> *"The souls of these noblest of blossoms could not be simply ripped from them; they had to be methodically coaxed away. In a special impregnating room, the flowers were strewn on glass plates, smeared with cool oil or wrapped in oil-soaked cloths; there they would die slowly in their sleep. It took three or four days for them to wither and exhale their scent into the adhering oil. Then they were carefully plucked off and new blossoms spread out. This procedure was repeated a good ten, twenty times, and it was September before the pomade had drunk its fill and the fragrant oil could be pressed from the cloths.*[3]

One difference between attars and other perfumes is that, in the Islamic tradition, alcohol is considered to destroy the soul of the plant, so although solvents are used in most perfumes (including absolutes), this is forbidden in attar manufacture. The Arabic word for alcohol (Al Khul) translates as body-eating spirit (also the origin of the word ghoul).

Attars give another dimension to healing and are a useful addition to a dispensary. They are used largely for their aroma, which has a great therapeutic effect. They are rarely used internally, but can be, with caution, in certain preparations.

Attars & the Olfactory System

"Smell is a potent wizard that transports us across a thousand miles and all the years we have lived."[4]

It has recently been found that certain odours trigger responses in the limbic system, which regulates mood and emotion, and affect both immune and nervous functions. This makes natural perfumes, attars, and resins a good alternative, or adjunct, to other natural healing tools, and are particularly useful when our right or ability to use herbal medicine is threatened.

Each nasal passage has a small (2.5 cm square) area containing fifty million sensory receptor cells, which send messages to the olfactory bulb (a projection of the brain). From the olfactory bulb, a signal is transmitted to the limbic system where memory is used to recognise odours.

Memory can be enhanced by certain smells, for example wild daffodil (nargis), lily of the valley, and frankincense can be used in cases of Alzheimer's and amnesia.

The limbic system also regulates mood and emotion.

Because attars are very pure (they contain no alcohol or solvents, which not only destroy the soul of the plant but spread its fragrance to those who may not want it), their perfume remains on the wearer's zone of intimacy.

Attars can be worn either on wrist points or in the ridge of the right ear (to directly influence nerve pathways).

Some attars contain more than forty pure ingredients and are secret family formulae; others can be traced directly to ancient healers or prophets.

Although primarily used in Unani Tibb medicine, attars are also used in Ayurveda, where they have a place in harmonising doshic or humoural imbalances.

The most popular botanical substances used in attar preparation include oudh, rose, saffron, jasmine, tuberose, amber, myrrh, sandalwood, and frankincense. Many of the secret Attari formulae may use as many as forty different essences, often including the rarest and most expensive perfumes, such as oudh (eaglewood), saffron (so expensive it is sold by the gram), and the finest rose petals (about thirty roses are required for just one drop of pure rose attar).

Many attars are manufactured to emulate, celebrate, or honour great people, places, occasions, or states of bliss. These are not blends, as in aromatherapy; in the Attari tradition, all ingredients are distilled together.

CHAPTER TWO

The Origins of Therapeutic Perfume

"Scent is life itself and, as breath, creates the world." [5]

Perhaps it was soon after the discovery of fire that we learned that certain barks, roots, flowers, and resins when heated or burned gave off an odour with particular properties, some narcotic, some toxic, some enhancing vision, others relaxing and healing.

Early Egyptian, Vedic, and Judaic texts, including the Ebers Papyrus, outline the use of many tree barks and resins used in ancient therapeutic perfumery.

The Ebers Papyrus (1550 BC) is thought to be the oldest document on herbs as medicine, and although it is predated by certain Vedic and Chinese texts, it is felt that the Ebers scroll was merely a copy of a much earlier document (around 2800 BC), which was considered to be the records of Thoth.[6]

The use of aromas in healing certainly dates back to around 2700 years BC to Imhotep, the Egyptian physician, magician, sage, and high priest to the sun god Ra. Imhotep was the architect of the Pyramid of Djoser and was described as "the one who comes in peace."

Imhotep wrote extensively on the treatment of more than two hundred diseases and was identified by the Greeks as Asclepius, the god of medicine and healing, and the founder of the healing tradition followed by Hippocrates.

Imhotep was known to recommend fragrances for bathing. These oils and resins (including frankincense, sandalwood, myrrh, and cinnamon) were also used to mummify the dead and often traded for gold.

Tapputi Belatekallin (Babylon 2000 BC) was one of the first perfumers and considered by some to be the first to develop the process of distillation. Tapputi used water, oil of balanos (taken from the desert date palm), calamus, cyperus,* myrrh, and balsam as the basis for many of her perfumes.

Evidence of the kind of distilling equipment used four thousand years ago (Bronze Age) was found in Pyrgos (Cyprus, the birthplace of Aphrodite), where a team of Italian archaeologists unearthed a perfume factory covering 4,000 square metres and containing at least sixty stills. The perfumes were kept in alabaster jars and included lavender, bay, laurel, myrtle, and pine. It is thought that the herbs were ground, added to oil and water, and buried in long-necked jugs over hot embers for twenty-four hours.[7]

Megallus (an ancient Greek perfumer) created a perfume known as megaleion, which contained cinnamon, myrrh, charred frankincense, and was steeped in oil of balanos. Megaleion was used for healing wounds and reducing inflammation.

Dioscorides used the ancient perfume oil known as metopian to draw out ulcers and treat cut sinews. Metopian was manufactured from bitter almond oil and unripe olives scented with cardamom, calamus, honey, wine, myrrh, galbanum, and turpentine resin.

Hippocrates, the father of modern medicine, used aromatic fumigation to rid Athens of the plague (as did the seer/herbalist Nostradamus two thousand years later in Northern Europe).

Aristotle (fourth century BC) was also thought to have invented the art of distillation, (an art later refined by the Arabs and Persians). Resins, woods, and flowers were steeped in oil (such as that taken from the balanites egyptiaca tree, plants of the moringa species, or castor, sesame, and sunflower).

Theophrastus (327–287 BC) wrote an essay entitled "On Odours."

HORUS FRAGRANCE: Going back before 2000 BC, "Seven Substances" were kept for the king in an unguent chamber for

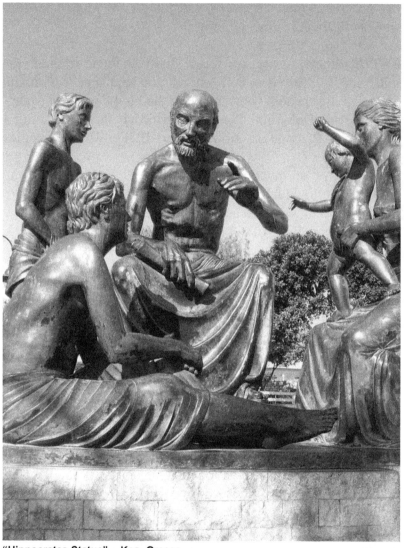

"Hippocrates Statue" - Kos, Greece

use in the hereafter. Excerpts from "The Magic Book on How to Prepare Unguents" were carved on the walls.

Earlier perfumes and unguents include such plants as cistus creticus (rockrose), lemongrass (camel grass), cardamom, calamus (sweet flag iris), cassia, cinnamon, cyperus (knotgrass), dill, henna (the perfume of henna was thought to be potent enough to resurrect the dead), iris, juniper, lily, lotus, saffron, spikenard, frankincense, and myrrh.

KYPHI: (kapet) an incense recipe that was found in the Pyramids and was used in both embalming and purification. Its formulation is generally attributed to the Egyptian priest Manetho ("Beloved of Thoth") who described it in a text entitled "Treatise on Preparation" (third century BC) of which no copies survive.

Kyphi is also mentioned in Dioscorides "Materia Medica" (AD 40–90) in which it is said to contain up to thirty-six key ingredients and was used as a potion, incense, and salve.

Ingredient lists of kyphi generally include spikenard, labdanum, cassia bark, cedar, cyperus, calamus, juniper, saffron, sandalwood, aloeswood, frankincense, styrax, mastic, benzoin, cardamom, galangal, lemongrass, rose petals, honey, raisins, and wine.

The kyphi recipe from the walls of the Ptolemaic Temple of Edfu lists carob, sugar, frankincense, styrax, calamus, mastic, violet, wine, and water.

According to Plutarch (AD second century), the formula includes raisins, honey, wine, myrrh, mastic, bitumen of Judea, cyperus,* juniper, calamus, and cardamom.

Other formulae contain various woods, including pine, oak, and palo santo.

Kyphi was used as an antidote to poisons, as a laxative, and to treat asthma-like conditions.

THERIAC/TYRIAC: Theriake (from the Greek for "wild beasts" or "poisonous reptiles"), a formula that has gone in and out of fashion for centuries, also uses many of the herbs and resins in kyphi with a great deal of saffron (in Avicenna's version).

---

*Cyperus longus (xiang fu, sweet nutgrass) is sometimes confused in translation as cypress (cuppressus species) and often galangal (the latter being in the same genus and often used in ancient incense and perfumes).

Avicenna refers a great deal to the compound theriaca (tiryaq) that was originally formulated in first century Greece. Theriaca became popular in China and India. The legendary history of theriaca begins with the compound mithridatium, supposedly formulated by King Mithridates VI (first century BC). King Mithridates was known to be immune to poisons. Mithridatium contained a high percentage of resins (including frankincense) together with saffron, cinnamon, and around thirty to fifty other herbs. This formula was modified and improved upon by Nero's physician, Andromachus, who brought the number of ingredients up to the alchemical number sixty-four and included viper flesh[8] (pit viper is still used today in Chinese medicine in the treatment of cancer and other "deep-seated" conditions). The Cabalist Moses ben Nahman lists the ingredients loosely as "leaven, honey, flesh of wild beasts and reptiles, dried scorpion, and viper."[9]

The Greek physician Galen devoted an entire book to theriaca and regularly prescribed it to Marcus Aurelius. The formula took years to gather and prepare, making it extremely expensive. Avicenna considered theriaca to be a general antidote to snake venom, poisons, and food toxins. This formula was used as a universal panacea until the eighteenth century, when it fell out of favour—it would now be considered (at least in Western countries) as not only illegal but also unethical.

Theriac was mentioned in Flaubert's *Madame Bovary.*

At least one highly modified theriaca formula does currently exist in the Western world, but it contains very few of the original ingredients.

Perfumes were oil-based until around AD 1150, when the use of alcohol (forbidden in Islam and in pure attar production) started to dominate.

CHYPRE: (French for cyprus) is loosely based on the above formulation. Chypre usually contains citron (citrus medica), labdanum (from cystus), oakmoss, styrax, and calamus. Some recipes include galbanum, patchouli, and bergamot.

CHISM: A consecrated oil made from rose, orange blossom, jasmine, cinnamon, benzoin, civet, musk, ambergris, and sesame oil. Chism has been used in the coronation of kings since the time of Charles the First (seventeenth century) and is still used today.

CHAPTER THREE

Natural Perfumes Used
in the Healing Traditions
of India, China, and Japan

Attars in Indian Ayurveda

"I am the sacred fragrance of the Earth" [10]

B *rihat Samhita* (AD 550), a major text of 105 chapters written by the sage Varahamihra, contains a chapter on the
manufacture of perfumes.

KHUS or VETIVERT is known in India as the Oil of Tranquillity, but it is also quite uplifting. Although it is cooling and
relaxing, it also helps to concentrate scattered thoughts.

Khus is a tonic and relaxant. It purifies the mind, blood, and
skin, is antiseptic, enhances concentration, purifies the mind,
cools anger, balances female hormones, and is an aphrodisiac.

Vetivert strengthens the nervous system. It reduces both
tension and depression while stabilizing energy. This deep, dark
perfume is a natural tranquillizer, being useful for insomnia, yet
(rather like many of the Asian adaptogens) it appears to possess
both sedative and stimulating properties.

Vetivert (khus) was mentioned in Atharvaveda and is linked
in yoga philosophy to the muladhara (root) chakra and therefore
good for treating fear, tremor, fatigue, and anxiety.

Vetivert is a tall grass with long aromatic roots from which
the oil is extracted by steam distillation. This herb has a long,

rich history and is considered one of the finest scents, having been used in perfumery for centuries.

LOTUS: (nelumbo nucifera)

Symbolism: "Expresses beauty above the mud of worldly concerns."

The lotus is probably the most important flower in both Indian and Egyptian mythology—both the Egyptian sun god (Ra) and the Vedic creator (Brahma) were born from the lotus. Studies have found that the lotus will germinate even after five hundred years in polluted ground. In the Vedic culture of India, the lotus is regarded as a sacred symbol of purity, peace, enlightenment, and beauty due to the observation of such a beautiful flower arising from often highly polluted waterways.

In ancient Hindu mythology, the lotus was said to spring from the navel of Vishnu (the maintainer) and seated within its petals was Brahma (the creator). A similar story comes from Ancient Egypt, where a child god was born from a giant blue lotus. The blue lotus was used to invoke Isis, Osiris, and Thoth.

Lotus (known as 'seshen') was also included in a recipe from the Edfu Temple and was used in sixteenth century Egypt to reduce fever.

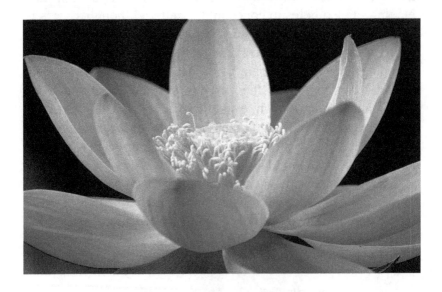

Saraswati, the consort of Brahma and goddess of wisdom, music, and the arts, is often depicted as sitting in a lotus—representing the crown chakra, the highest seat of consciousness.

SANDALWOOD: "The mother of all attars," is heralded by all traditions and has been used for more than four thousand years throughout the world. Sandalwood was given royal status in 1792 by the Sultan of Mysore, resulting in the Indian government being the official owner of all sandalwood trees in India. The best sandalwood is said to come from Mysore and Tamil Nadu, although the tree does grow in Australia and several Arabic countries.

In India, sandalwood oils and incenses are used to calm the mind for meditation, and it is not uncommon to see forest sadhus (holy men) wearing not only sandalwood rosaries but also sandalwood paste on the brow to cool the brain. As a cosmetic preparation, sandalwood assists in reducing wrinkles.

Medicinal uses: Sandalwood is used to treat digestive disorders, as a muscle relaxant, to treat skin problems, stress, and depression. Sandalwood is a tonic sedative and used by spiritual traditions to promote compassion.

Sandalwood has antidepressant, nervine, sedative, and tranquilizing properties; it enhances concentration, is antispasmodic, anti-inflammatory, antibacterial, antipyretic, diuretic, and relieves burning and itching of the urinary tract.

Sandalwood oils and attars are becoming much more expensive due to their endangered status, and although cheaper oils are available throughout the Arab world, they are not as potent as those from Mysore.

The above three attars work well together, as all have a relaxing element. Lotus is a floral, higher-note perfume, sandalwood is woody, middle to bottom, and vetivert is resinous and deep.

Other major attars used in Indian Ayurveda

CHAMPA (michellia champaca): Promotes circulation, elevates moods, releases emotions, enhances romantic feelings, and is a decongestant.

Green champa is considered to be cooling—it is known as "The Cobra Type," as it seems to attract snakes. Yellow champa is more warming.[11]

HINA (henna flower, lawsonia inermis): Strengthens mind and body, rejuvenates, enhances circulation, and is an alterative nervine tonic and tranquilizer.

Hina is thought to open the third Chakra and to awaken Kundalini.

"The lord of sweet-smelling blossoms in this world and the next" [12]

"The scent of this herb was reputed to resurrect the dead." [13]

JASMINE: Is an antidepressant, antibacterial, enhances memory, an aphrodisiac, and is thought to balance the three Doshas* and support harmony in the five elements.

PATCHOULI: Calms the mind, is an antidepressant, antibacterial, antiseptic, a mild aphrodisiac, memory stimulant, and is grounding.

ROSE: "Queen of Flowers" is romantic, an aphrodisiac, mild laxative, antidepressant, and promotes immunity.

SAFFRON: Blood cleanser, improves colour of complexion, enhances clarity of perception, decongestant, aphrodisiac, balances hormones, and is rich in quercetin.

Attars for harmonizing specific doshas (body types) in Ayurveda

VATA: (Air/Ether)—warming, calming oils, including cedar, frankincense, jasmine, orange, sandalwood, and lotus. Hina: specific for vata-type pain. Vetivert recreates lost harmony.

---

*The three doshas in Ayurvedic medicine are:
Vata: combines the elements of air and ether.
Pitta: refers to fire and water.
Kapha: earth and water.
These are constitutional types. They are often found in combination and are affected by time, season, and situation.

PITTA: (Fire/Water)—cooling, sweet-smelling oils, include rose, sandalwood, mint, myrrh, frankincense, gardenia, and vetivert (khus).

Khus: (the oil of tranquillity) is specific for pitta headache.

Sandalwood: Pitta headache, inflammation, burning.

KAPHA: (Earth/Water)—invigorating, opening, warming, includes juniper, pine, cinnamon, frankincense, and myrrh.

* * *

Fragrance in China

From the third or fourth century BC in China, the Taoist tradition has revered the use of incense, believing that every perfume is a medicine and that the extraction of fragrance from a plant actually liberates the plant's soul. The transformation of solid incense into smoke or vapour represents and mirrors the transmutation that takes place from the physical to the spiritual realms.

Functions of attars relating to Chinese medicine

ATLAS CEDAR: Is used for nourishing kidney yin and calming "shen" (heart/spirit). It nourishes kidney and bladder qi (energy) deficiency, resolves phlegm, and invigorates blood (varicosis). Cedar is used in Tibet to treat bronchial and urinary infections and to calm the mind.

MANDARIN/ORANGE PEEL/NEROLI: Moves liver qi (with jasmine), harmonises shen,* and aids digestion.

PALMAROSA: Is thought to tonify heart blood and qi deficiency with shen weakness. It strengthens the spleen and regulates digestion.

PATCHOULI: Nourishes heart and kidney yin (with vetivert, rose, neroli, and myrrh); strengthens spleen, resolving toxic damp, abdominal bloating (with palmarosa and vetivert); invigorates blood in lower limbs. Patchouli can be used for pain and insomnia and acts as an insect repellent.

SANDALWOOD: is one of the great "xiang" remedies and is known in China as "Tan xiang" and parallels with rosewood ("jiang xiang"), aloeswood ("Chen xiang"), and frankincense ("Ru xiang").

VETIVERT (KHUS): Nourishes blood and essence, regulates menstruation and menopause; nourishes yin (yin deficiency with empty heat), calms shen (with spikenard and patchouli); strengthens the spleen (with patchouli and palmarosa); dispels wind-damp heat, relaxes tendons, and relieves pain.

In Chinese terms, khus nourishes blood, yin, and essence, clears heat, and calms shen.*

YLANG YLANG: Spreads liver qi, harmonizes shen (when combined with rose, jasmine, atlas cedar, helps with shock and extreme trauma); harmonizes liver and spleen, and lifts depression (with jasmine); nourishes liver and heart blood.

Much of the above functions are drawn from the work of Peter Holmes, who has applied a Chinese energetic approach to fragrances.

Holmes P. *Aromatica, A Clinical Guide to Essential Oil Therapeutics; Volume 1 Principles and Profiles. 2016. + Volume 2. Applications and Profiles.* 2019. Singing Dragon, London and Philadelphia.

Other terms referring to Chinese medicine include qi, which refers loosely to energy, either within or outside of the body; and as used in martial arts—Qi Gong, Tai Chi, etc. There are three major types of qi referred to in traditional Chinese medicine: 1. Ancestral Qi, relating to the kidneys and adrenals; 2. Acquired Qi, relating to stomach and spleen; 3. Protective Qi, primarily lung.

YIN AND YANG: Yin tends to refer to internal energy and yang to expressed energy—traditionally described as 'the shady side of the mountain' (yin), and 'the sunny side of the mountain'

---

*Shen refers to heart or spirit essence. This is a term largely synonymous with "Ruh" (breath, spirit) in Arabic.

(yang)—they are not opposites, merely two sides of the same coin. In the words of George Oshawa, "everything that has a front, has a back."

The writings of Confucius included references to the importance of fragrance; he was particularly fond of orchids, which he saw as a symbol of noble character. The orchid has been cultivated in China for more than two thousand years.

"If you are in the company of good people, it is like entering a room full of orchids. After a while, you become soaked in the fragrance and you don't even notice it. If you are in the company of bad people, it is like going into a room that smells of fish. After a while, you don't notice the fishy smell as you have been immersed in it." [14]

* * *

Japan: (the Way of Incense)

In Japan the term "*Kodo*" means "The Way of Incense" and (like the term attar) incense is translated as fragrance.

The first formal record of incense in Japan was 595 CE and relates to the discovery of a log of agarwood that floated ashore on a Japanese island.

Samurai warriors were known to purify themselves with incense before going into battle.

Incense/fragrance in Japan was known to purify, sharpen the senses, calm and awaken the spirit.

Ingredients used included agarwood, sandalwood, patchouli, spikenard, lily, and safflower.

CHAPTER FOUR

Herbal Medicine—as Old as the Ark

The Old Testament[15] tells how Moses was instructed to build the Ark of the Covenant with shittim wood—known to be a species of acacia—a tree with many uses.

Acacia (Australian wattle) is used by Australian aborigines to make boomerangs.

The smoke of acacia wood is thought (in the Tibetan tradition) to keep away demons and ghosts.

Acacia seeds are used in Burma, Laos, and Thailand as a food and included in soups, omelettes, stir-fries, and curries.

The acacia tree is used as a symbol of Freemasonry.

Acacia Senegal is used in the production of gum arabic.

Acacia is thought by many to be the Burning Bush cited in Exodus.

More than ten species of acacia are used in perfumery.

Acacia root has been used for stomach cancer, rheumatoid arthritis, depression, nervous exhaustion, and stress-related conditions.[16]

A related species, albizzia julibrissin (Persian silk tree), is described as the tree of happiness by the Chinese and was first documented in the AD second century for its calming properties.[17]

Albizzia is recommended by the American master herbalist Michael Tierra to relieve anxiety, stress, and depression. It contains several compounds of flavonol glycosides, which have demonstrated sedative activity.[18]

Hermes (in some cultures referred to as a legendary god, by others as the founder of alchemy and a contemporary of Moses) was thought to be the first to use perfumes in healing. These

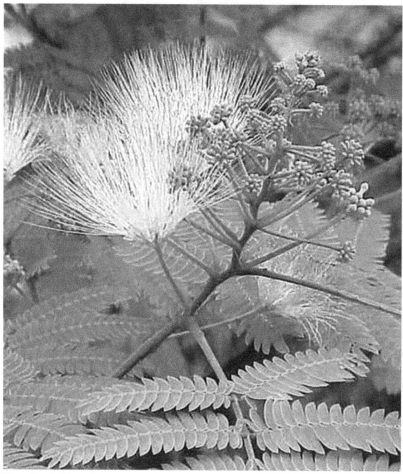

"Persian Silk Tree"

formulations were used by ancient Egyptian, Greek, Roman, and Middle Eastern traditions (also in the earliest records of Indian Ayurvedic medicine).

History records many of the valuable essences made from florals, resins, and barks that were used by Cleopatra, the Queen of Sheba, Mohammed, Dioscorides, and many others. Biblical importance is attached to frankincense, myrrh, aloeswood, and other incenses used, not only at the birth of Christ, but also by Moses in the Ark of the Covenant, which was buried in a chamber beneath the first Temple of Solomon in Jerusalem. (The Ark is now reputed to exist in one of several locations, including a small temple in Ethiopia and the Qu'aba in Mecca.)

> *And the* LORD *said unto Moses, "Take unto thee sweet spices, stacte, and onycha, and galbanum; these sweet spices with pure frankincense: of each shall there be a like weight: And thou shalt make it a perfume, a confection after the art of the apothecary, tempered together, pure and holy."[19]*

(It is interesting to note that this incense formula used in the Ark of the Covenant incorporates top (head), middle (heart), and base notes, as with modern perfumery.)

STACTE: (styrax, storax, Turkish sweetgum, liquidambar orientalis) is thought to have originated from Syria or the Levant. Stacte provides a middle or heart note to the above formula.

According to Herodotus (440 BC) styrax resin was burned as an incense to drive away winged serpents, which were said to protect the frankincense trees.

Avicenna (AD tenth century) refers to styrax as a dental restorative; it has antibacterial and disinfectant properties; it soothes the lungs and bronchi (it is actually used as an additive by tobacco companies).

ONYCHA: There are many translations for this word. The Torah refer to it as a mollusc shell or the mucous door of the onyx snail. Some sources claim it to be costus root (aucklandia lappa) or even spikenard (nardostachys jatamansi). Onycha is the base note in this formula and generally considered to be labdanum, a resin taken from cistus creticus.

GALBANUM: (ferula gummosa, giant fennel, sacred mother resin). This giant fennel grows mainly in Northern Persia (Iran). Galbanum provides a top note to the formula; its resin belongs to the green family of scents. Legend states that the torch used by Prometheus to bring fire to humanity was made from the stem of a giant fennel.

This potent plant is used in Coptic medicine to protect against snakes and insects. Dioscorides also used it as a sedative and analgesic. It can also be used to treat boils and aching muscles.

A more modern use of this green top note is in Chanel No. 19 by Coco Chanel.

QETORET: (ketoret, Solomon's incense) was said by the mediaeval Sephardic Jewish philosopher Maimonides to contain eleven ingredients, including the above three (stacte, onycha, and galbanum); the other eight were thought to be myrrh, deer musk, cassia, nard, saffron, costus, aromatic bark (possibly from the frankincense tree), and cinnamon.

Solomon himself was known for his references to several herbs and resins:

"All thy garments smell of myrrh, and aloes, and cassia . . ." [20]

"Your plants are a paradise of pomegranates with the fruits of the orchard; cypress with spikenard, spikenard and saffron, sweet cane and cinnamon, with all the trees of Libanus, myrrh and aloes with all the chief perfumes." [21]

"Spikenard and saffron; calamus and cinnamon, with all trees of frankincense, myrrh and aloes, with all the chief spices." [22]

Aloes (referred to in the above quotes from the Song of Solomon) is generally considered to be "oudh" (otherwise known as aloeswood or agarwood), a tree from the aquilaria species.

"The sweet odour of the tree of life shall enter into the bones of the chosen and they shall live a long life." [23]

* * *

The Gifts of the Magi

So, who were the Magi? Some say they came from a Persian priestly caste that paid great attention to the stars. Some say that they were Zoroastrian astrologer priests from Babylon who believed that Jesus was the great leader prophesied in the Old Testament (Micah 5:2). Others claim they came from different

21

regions and met along the Silk Route on their way to Israel (their names have Persian, Phoenician, and Yemeni origins). In their travels they might have passed through countries such as Iraq, Saudi Arabia, Syria, Turkey, Cyprus, and Greece (Crete), to name just a few. They may have brought their treasures from their homeland or sought them along the way. These gifts were said to be symbolic of kingship (gold), priesthood (frankincense), death and resurrection (myrrh).

GOLD: Apart from being a rare and precious metal, gold has always been used as a medicine. From the monatomic substances (Mfkzt) allegedly fed to ancient pharaohs, to the gold *bhasmas* (alchemically prepared ashes) used in Ayurvedic medicine, to the gold salts currently used in the treatment of arthritis, to the gold compounds being researched as potential cancer cures, gold has a potent place in the history of medicine. But gold is rarely (if ever) used in perfumes (apart from the exquisite bottles sometimes found in the East). So for the purpose of this book, I will give more space to frankincense and myrrh.

FRANKINCENSE: The frankincense tree has always been valued throughout the Middle and Far East. The word for the sap from this beautiful tree is synonymous with the Arabic word for milk (*al lubn*), which gave rise to the name Lebanon, whose mountains are always capped with milk-white snow. Frankincense resin is one of the oldest true (frank) incenses and one of the most expensive commodities traded throughout the East. Like so many precious plant substances, frankincense trees were said to be protected by fierce bats and snakes and grown in dangerous, inaccessible regions; this and the dangers involved in carrying the resin throughout the Silk Route and other difficult passes kept the price high and the traders rich.

There are more than fifty biblical references to frankincense. This precious resin was significant to the birth (and death) of Christ. Frankincense (*ru xiang*) is used in Chinese medicine to invigorate blood and reduce swelling. In Islamic medicine, it is used with sandalwood "to carry the soul to heaven."

Frankincense is used in inhalation as an analgesic and traditionally used in Eastern attars to protect against malevolent influences. The pure resin can be taken internally (often ground with coffee, to treat amnesia). It is a major attar in enlivening memory and may be useful in treating Alzheimer's.

Research on frankincense is underway for arthritic conditions, low back pain, fibrositis, colitis, Crohn's disease, and asthma.

The best frankincense (*hougari*) comes from Oman, where immunologist Mahmoud Suhail is hoping to open a new chapter in its history: Scientists have observed that there is some agent within frankincense that stops cancer from spreading and induces cancerous cells to close themselves down. He is trying to find out what that agent is.

"Cancer starts when the DNA code within the cell's nucleus becomes corrupted," he says. "It seems frankincense has a re-set function. It can tell the cell what the right DNA code should be. Frankincense separates the 'brain' of the cancerous cell—the nucleus—from the 'body'—the cytoplasm, and closes down the nucleus to stop it reproducing corrupted DNA codes." [24]

(Chemotherapy works by destroying the tissue around a tumour to kill the cancer but will also destroy healthy cells.)

MYRRH: Myrrh is also a highly protective herb and is used as a resin, tincture, or perfume attar for its antiviral, anti-infection, antibacterial, antiseptic, astringent, carminative, and anti-inflammatory properties.

Myrrh was traditionally burned around a woman giving birth to protect against postpartum infections; the newborn child was then fumigated with the smoke of the burned resin for forty days.

Myrrh was mentioned in ancient Egyptian texts (2,800 BC) as sacred to Isis. It is one of the ingredients in the ancient incense kyphi and the ointment metopium used for treating infected wounds.

There are various sources of myrrh—one is synonymous with the biblical *labdanum* derived from the cistus (rockrose) of Crete, Cyprus, and North Africa. Labdanum resin was traditionally gathered from the flanks and beards of the goats that grazed among the cistus shrubs. It is now gathered with a rake-like tool known as a labdanisterion.

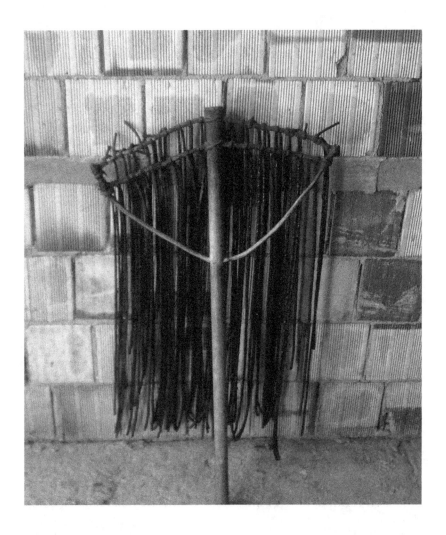

Labdanum resin has a perfume reminiscent of ambergris and is often combined with frankincense, mastic, and other resins in ancient healing salves.

Labdanum (ladan) was also an ingredient in an ancient incense recipe (known as kyphi) found in the Pyramids. The recipe was said to contain up to thirty-six ingredients and used both as a potion and a salve.

Chypre (French for cypress) is also a blend of resins containing labdanum, oak moss, storax, and calamus.

Another form of myrrh, commonly used in Ayurvedic medicine, is guggul (commifora mukul—common myrrh).

The myrrh resin is usually combined with other herbs to make it more bioavailable (guggul should not be taken in its raw form but only in accepted preparations). Guggul is used to treat obesity, relieve arthritis (having anti-inflammatory and pain-relieving properties), to lower cholesterol,[25] harmonise blood pressure, and protect against hardening of the arteries. Guggul also improves immune function by increasing the production of red blood cells and improving the activity of white blood cells.

As a blood purifier, guggul can be helpful in correcting skin disorders such as eczema.

Clinical studies on the use of guggul in the above conditions have been positive.

In Ayurvedic medicine, guggul is classified as a *rasayana* (elixir) and recommended for all conditions affected by the ageing process.

Both frankincense and myrrh have been prized in the past as more valuable than gold.

According to ancient myths, both were sacred to the gods and protected by venomous snakes and vampire bats.

This article was first published (in part) by *Inspired Times* UK.

CHAPTER FIVE

The Persian Tradition

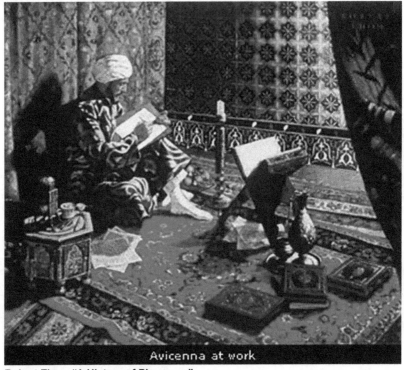

Avicenna at work

Robert Thom "A History of Pharmacy"

Avicenna (Ibn Sina) was a tenth century Persian physician, mystic, and alchemist who wrote almost three hundred learned texts on various subjects, including medicine, philosophy, astronomy, and religion. His fourteen-volume text *The Canon of Medicine* influenced medical thought for a thousand years, until the time of Edward Jenner, Louis Pasteur, and others whose focus was more about targeting infections and bacteria rather than treating the whole person.

Avicenna came from a small town near Bokhara in what is now Uzbekistan (and was then part of Greater Persia). Bokhara was central to the Silk Route (whose caravans were largely financed by Uzbek Jews). This route was used by Greek and Turkish scholars of the healing traditions of Hippocrates and Galen who travelled East in search of new medicines and new knowledge. From China, Tibet, and India came the Ayurvedic Vedyas, Chinese and Tibetan alchemists, and the merchants trading in silks, gems, and other commodities. A stopping-off place for many of these travellers was Bagdad, which was one of the world's great centres of discourse and learning.

Avicenna learned from some of the greatest minds of both East and West and added medicines and skills to his treasure chest from natural healing traditions, resulting in him becoming the chief physician of the royal court of Persia at a very early age.

Avicenna was known to be the first to distil roses. He included no less than sixty attars (perfume essences) in his pharmacopoeia of cardiac tonics. He considered that, "The vital power of the heart is attracted to aromas."

Of the sixty-three cardiac medicines mentioned by Avicenna, forty were aromatic oils (attars). They included lavender, rose, cinnamon, frankincense, water lily or lotus, mint, aloeswood, saffron, and basil.

Disorders caused by coldness were treated with warming attars such as musk, amber, saffron, aloeswood, and cardamom. Cooling attars include camphor, sandalwood, rose, and coriander.

The alchemist Jabir and the nature doctors Rhazes and Avicenna (Ibn Sina) brought together knowledge and medicines from the greatest traditions, including Greece, Babylon, Arabia, Egypt, and Indochina. The ancient Persian Empire (600–343 BC) had spanned a huge tract of land from parts of Greece to the border with India. The Persia of the Islamic period (from AD ninth century), which was the birthplace of both Rhazes and Ibn Sina (Bokhara—then in Afghanistan—now in Uzbekistan), was conveniently placed in the central point of the Great Silk Route, bringing merchants, philosophers, and mendicants from

West to East and East to West—this trade was largely financed by the Jews of Bokhara. Much of this knowledge condensed in the Abbasid capital Baghdad.

History tells us that the Caliph of Baghdad, Harum al-Rashid (largely responsible for the Arabian Nights—with the help of Scheherazade), dreamed he was visited by Aristotle and was inspired to have Aristotle's writings translated into Arabic; these were followed by the writings of Hippocrates and other luminaries. Much of the translations were made by Christians, who were among the polyglot of cultures still living in the Middle East in this period.

Unani Tibb was inspired by the physicians Rhazes and Avicenna in the ninth and tenth centuries, and the earlier influences of Hippocrates and Galen are clear to see.

This system was further developed in the tenth century by the Persian physician Hakim Ibn Sina (known in the west as Avicenna). Avicenna compiled the classic text *The Canon of Medicine,* which influenced both the teaching and practice of medicine for the next thousand years.

Literally translated as *Greek Medicine,* Unani Tibb was influenced by the teachings of Hippocrates (circa 500 BCE) but also incorporates much of the healing arts of China, India, Tibet, and the Middle East.

Avicenna was also known for his development and use of attars to treat many disorders, particularly those associated with the heart, emotions, and the evolution of the soul (*Ruh*), adding to a range of exhilarants and nervines unequalled by other traditional medicine systems.

Ibn Sina (Avicenna) wrote more than two hundred works, including *The Canon of Medicine*, a five-volume text, which influenced medicine for more than 800 years (up until the time of Louis Pasteur and others who considered that the aim of medicine was not to create a state of wholeness and balance but to protect against "external evils").

Many teachings of Ibn Sina also influenced the work of later Sufi mystics, poets, philosophers, and physicians including Attari,[26] Rumi, and Hafiz.

Unani Tibb medicine is based on three important concepts:

The Theory of Naturals—indicates how deviation from a state of balance gives rise to disease.

The Doctrine of Causes—explains the reason behind this deviation.

The Doctrine of Signs—concerning diagnostic procedures.

Among the theories of Unani Tibb are Tabiat, described as a mysterious power that all living beings have access to and which maintains good health.

The theory of Tabiat was laid down by Hippocrates in his teaching: "*Nature heals; the physician is only nature's assistant.*"

Unani Tibb is, of course, a vast subject and it is not my aim in this article to outline even its key principles, but a particular interest of mine involves Ibn Sina's healing approach based on sense of smell. As the first person to distil roses, he recognised that attars (pure perfumes) are a fast and powerful way of treating the soul/spirit, which in many traditions was connected to the heart.[27]

Ibn Sina was best known as a heart doctor and up to forty of his more than sixty prescriptions for the heart were actually perfumes,[28] ranging from single-plant extractions to complex combinations distilled together.

Ibn Sina felt that the vital power of the heart is attracted to aromas and once remarked, "All aromatic oils are cardiac drugs."

Many other uses of attars are cited in Ibn Sina's *The Canon of Medicine*, including:

On exposure to heat: "one should use oil of rose and violets on the journey, anointing the back with them from time to time." [29]

Remedy for excessive purgation: "should also be invigorated by the use of fragrant perfumes."[30]

Attars were also commonly recommended at that time "to attract angels" and "ward off evil spirits" (the word "ward," often used as a protective spell, is also an Arabic word for rose).

Among the attars (non-alcoholic distilled plant essences) used by Ibn Sina were rose (described by Hakim Sherif of Kabul as "Queen of the Garden of Paradise"), and frankincense (now being researched as a potential cure for everything from Alzheimer's to cancer).[31]

More complex distillations of multiple plants evolved to emulate certain states or "Stations of the Soul,"* including "Nafs Mutamainah" (Settled Soul), "Shafaya'at" (The Healer), and "Jannat al-Ferdous (Gateway to the Highest Paradise).

The use of attars in healing can be instrumental in treating many of the underlying causes of ill health. In a time of herbal regulation, endangered plants, and problems regarding access to many herbs and formulae, attars could play an important role in the health practitioner's pharmacy.

Each of these stations relate to different physical and spiritual conditions (apart from the sixth station, which is free from all physical and spiritual conditions), and each station will respond to different fragrances or attars.

---

*In Unani philosophy, there are believed to be six stations of the evolution of the soul. They are: 1. the station of the ego (*Maqam am Nafs*); 2. the station of the heart (*Maqam al Qalb*); 3. the station of the soul (*Maqam al Ruh*); 4. the station of divine secrets (*Maqam as Sur*); 5. the station of nearness (*Maqam al Qurb*); and 6. the station of oneness or divine union (*Maqam al Wisal*).

CHAPTER SIX

Attars of Arabia

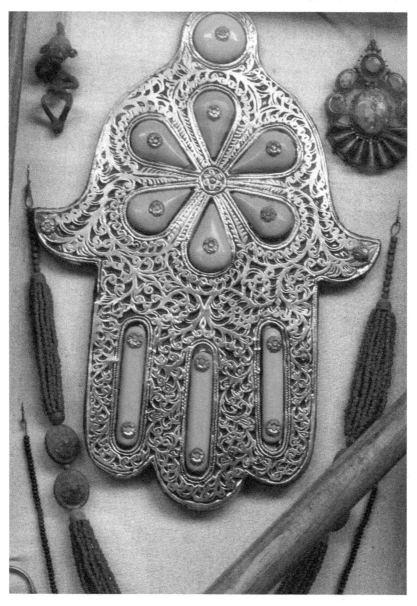

FRANKINCENSE: (boswellia sacra, boswellia carteri) "franc encens" (lit. pure incense)

"Use frankincense for it invigorates the heart with courage and it is a remedy for forgetfulness." [32]

"Fumigate your house with olibanum and thyme."[33] Frankincense dispels malevolent and distressing psychic forces, improves memory, and cleanses the aura. Frankincense was used to ward off negativity (exorcism), and pestilence.

Frankincense was favoured by Mohammed, who added the resin to his coffee to increase alertness.

Frankincense is antidepressant, anti-inflammatory, analgesic. It tonifies heart and lung qi with shen weakness, resolves phlegm, and dispels wind/damp.

Frankincense was traditionally charred and used as eyeliner to ward off the evil eye.

Frankincense was once a key merchandise traded between Rome, Greece, Arabia, China, and India.

Pliny recorded that huge amounts were burned by Emperor Nero at the last rites for his departed wife.

Some of the best frankincense (hougari) comes from Oman, where it is burned at all festive events. Burned frankincense is a major ingredient in kohl (used as an eye shadow in Eastern countries).

The bark of the frankincense tree (in the pine family) can be used, as can the resin. Frankincense oils and attars are also available.

In ancient times the gathering of frankincense was an inherited privilege, and those gathering the resin maintained both celibacy and avoided attending funerals.

JASMINE: (chameli, sien hing hwa, yasmin. Queen of the Night, Gift of God.) The word yasmine (Arabic) means fragrant oil.

* * *

Travelling through the mountains and gorges of Southwest Crete, we came to a small harbour town where we took a room in a taverna.

That evening I became aware of the beautiful smell of the night-flowering jasmine cladding the sides of the building. I thought that there must be somewhere in Crete where I could buy a good attar of this scent. In spite of much shopping around, it wasn't until the day we were leaving the island that I hurriedly bought a small bottle of jasmine from a woman in the backstreet markets of Heraklion.

When we had boarded the plane to return home, I opened the bottle and realized I should have bought more, as this was quite special.

On subsequent trips to Heraklion I bought further small amounts from this person, but she never had more than a bottle or two to sell.

Jasmine is the symbolic flower of Damascus and the national flower of Pakistan.

It is used in Chinese medicine for its aphrodisiac, calming, antibacterial, astringent, and antitumour properties. Jasmine is best known as an important source of natural perfume.

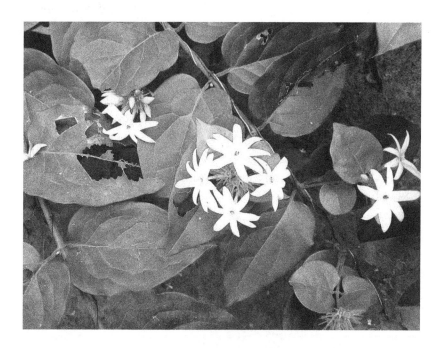

In the Chinese Song Dynasty (AD ninth century), the emperor insisted on having several hundred pots of Arabian jasmine in his courtyard. It is also reputed that Cleopatra favoured this perfume.

Jasmine oils are often chemically extracted with the use of solvents, whereas attars are either stone rolled, steam distilled (with sandalwood oil), or the flowers are pressed with olive oil between glass or gauze frames (the flowers are changed many times). It takes approximately eight hundred kilos of flowers to produce one kilo of high-quality attar.

The mystic whirling dervishes of Turkey favour jasmine. It uplifts moods and lessens depression.

Jasmine is good to be worn in the presence of children and generally around the home for pleasant dreams.

Properties: calmative, antidepressant, aphrodisiac, uplifting yet relaxing, uplifting moods and relieving depression, "dives deep into the soul," nourishes tissues, strengthens the nervous system, promotes emotional security, relieves shock and trauma, nourishes heart and liver blood, and regulates menses. Jasmine is mildly narcotic.

Jasmine is my attar of choice for supporting the emotions.

Jasmine has been used to treat epilepsy and stage fright.

This attar is "unparalleled in its ability to lessen depression,"—Hakim Chishti.

Jasmine has been hailed by German scientists to be as powerfully effective as Valium.[34] NHS choices (July 12, 2010).

Jasmine is "tridoshic" as it benefits all body types; it is thought to nourish both bodily tissues (when used in Marma therapy), and its perfume is thought to nourish the nervous system. Jasmine is cooling, antibacterial, aphrodisiac, antidepressant, and enhances memory.

CHAPTER SEVEN

Sacred Scents

66 **A** good friend and a bad friend are like a perfume seller and a blacksmith; the perfume seller might give you some perfume as a gift, or you might buy some from him, or at least you might smell its fragrance.

As for the blacksmith, he might burn your clothes, and at the very least you will breathe in the fumes of the furnace." [35]

SAFFRON: (zaffran, kesari, za'faran, krokos "bringer of good fortune"). Saffron is considered to be more valuable than gold by the ounce—it takes 4,000 stigmas from the pale purple crocus to make one ounce of pure saffron.

Saffron has also been used to treat cancer. In 1997, an herbal compound for cancer was patented; the original formula appeared in Avicenna's *The Canon of Medicine* in the tenth century. It was given the name *Hindiba* and appears to be based on the herb saffron.

Saffron is used as a powerful medicine in many traditions to treat spiritual, mental, and physical imbalances. It is said to nourish the heart, heighten the spirit, benefit insomnia, aid digestion, act as a sedative, rejuvenate, relieve depression, stimulate menses, and ease labour.

Saffron can be used in the treatment of eye infections, corneal disease, cataracts, pain, ulcers, open wounds, throat inflammation, and genital ulcers.[36]

Saffron is also recommended in cases of dyspnoea, painful urination, childbirth, menstrual disorders, and diseases of the head—*Assyrian Dictionary of Botany* circa 668-633 BCE.

Gerard recommends its use for plague and smallpox. The Black Death gave rise to an increase in saffron use.

Saffron is taken from the tiny stamens of the crocus flower, unfortunately the cheap 'saffron' sold in Middle Eastern tourist resorts is usually safflower, which possesses many of saffron's properties but is much milder in action. It is generally thought that the best true saffron comes from Kashmir and Iran; however, others have a high regard for Spanish "Mancha" saffron. A favourite of mine is sourced from the high Atlas Mountains in Morocco.

Perfume/Attar: To prepare a perfume, saffron stamens are stone rolled in sandalwood oil—the result has a mildly medicinal fragrance and is said to "release the transcendent essences of childhood."[37]

Wild about Saffron

It was more than forty years ago when I awoke one morning to a view across the Kashmir Valley. In the far distance, Dhal Lake shimmered in the morning sun, and to my left the mountain peaks glistened with snow. Before me lay fields of purple and gold—it was saffron season. Little did I realize that in my later life as an herbalist I would come to respect this herb as one which crosses over the manmade boundaries between body, mind, and spirit.

Let's start, as with all good stories, at the beginning—fifty thousand years ago in Mesopotamia with the early cave artist/ hunters. What did they use as a yellow pigment to colour their subjects on cave walls? You've got it—saffron!

If we jump forward a few millennia to the time of Cleopatra, what (amongst other things) did this great queen use in her bath? Yes, saffron! (Golden skin was in vogue at that time, as it was with early Buddhists, who didn't draw the line at yellow robes but also used saffron to colour their skin in emulation of the golden Buddha.)

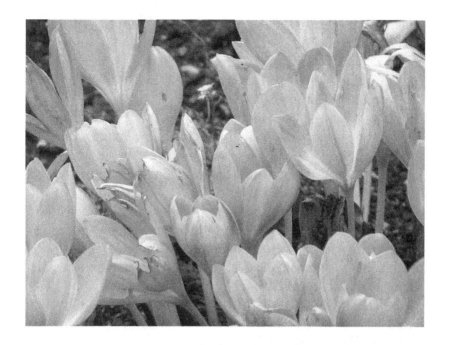

Early Phoenicians dedicated saffron to the goddess Astarte and used it as a treatment for melancholy.

An Indian legend states that saffron (*kesari*) was given to the physician Waghbatta by a water serpent god to cure the god's eye infection.

Saffron is mentioned in Shen Nong's great herbal *The Pen Ts'ao* (circa 200 BC) and in The Song of Solomon.

Saffron *(za'fran)* was sacred to the Egyptian god Amen.

Legend tells how Hermes created saffron when he accidentally wounded his friend Crocus.

The streets of Rome were strewn with saffron when Nero entered the city.

In Germany, saffron was used to ward off the plague, and the crime of adulterating saffron for sale was punishable by death.

In Switzerland, saffron is still used in protective amulets.

La Mancha saffron from a particular area of Spain has gained protective status.

Cultivation: It is believed that the earliest cultivation of saffron was near the southern Turkish town of Colysus, from which the name 'crocus' was supposedly derived. Historical documents report that saffron was brought into Kashmir from Persia around 500 BC.

The cultivation of saffron in England (Saffron Walden) was encouraged by Edward VII.

Preparation: It takes around 150,000 flowers to make one kilogram of saffron—190 flowers to make one gram.

The stigmas of crocus sativa produce the purest saffron (Mogra Zafran), whereas the stamens (Lacha Zafran) are less expensive and considered inferior.

Medicinal Properties: Saffron is used as a culinary herb, a colouring agent, and a medicine to treat depression. It is said to nourish the heart, heighten the spirit, benefit insomnia, aid digestion (carminative), act as a sedative, rejuvenative and antidepressant, stimulate menses (emmenagogue), and ease labour.

Saffron was an ingredient in the formula *Theriaca,* which was based on the compound *Mithridatium*, supposedly formulated by King Mithridates VI (first century BC).

Galen devoted an entire volume to Theriaca and regularly prescribed it to Marcus Aurelius. The formula took years to prepare and was extremely expensive—its use, however, survived until the eighteenth century.

Perfume/Attar: To prepare a perfume, saffron stamens are stone rolled in sandalwood oil before distillation.

Alchemical Properties: Saffron is referred to as the gold of the plant kingdom. It relates to the fire element and is ruled by Jupiter. Saffron is believed by alchemists to carry the signature of the transmuting agent.

Yoga/Ayurveda: In Indian medicine, saffron is considered to be pure *sattva* (the element of spiritual and etheric energy) and is used to clear and purify the *nadis* (subtle energy channels).

Back to the kitchen: Take one teaspoon of best saffron (you are worth it), place in a Pyrex bowl and cover with two cups of boiling water. Leave in the sun to cool for a few minutes (just to enjoy the colour produced). Pour half into a glass, add a little honey, and drink. Strain the other half over a cup of white basmati rice, leave to soak before adding more water and cooking. The strained-off herb can be used again for a milder infusion later.

* * *

OUDH: (agarwood, aloeswood, aquilaria, eaglewood, chien hsiang, jinkoh). The most-sought-after attar, traded by mystics and alchemists throughout the East. Oudh is considered by dervishes to be one of the greatest medicines for the mind and spirit.

The resin taken from this tree is said to be produced as a natural immune response to parasitic attacks (philaphora parasitica) and therefore only found in infected trees. As a result, oudh is rare, expensive, highly cherished, and traded amongst Unani, Ayurvedic, and Chinese healers, exotic oil traders, alchemists, and religious leaders. The best oudh comes from older trees.

The perfume of oudh attars can vary from a rich, almost faecal smell to sweeter, spicier fragrances.

Traditional Uses: Stimulant, cardio tonic, calmative, eases pain, antimicrobial, aphrodisiac, useful for lung disorders, including asthma and TB, calms and nourishes the heart.

The Prophet Muhammad stated that oudh contains the cure for seven diseases, and as a result it is used to perfume the cloth covering the Holy Qu'Aba in Mecca.

"Pure Oudh is unbelievable—it's an infection of the acquiver tree in India,* in response to the fungus, the tree creates an incredible dense amber** resin that smells of mould, sweet decaying wood, vivid green notes.

Most people hate it when they first encounter it and yet it seeds itself in your imagination—becomes addictive. These darker notes are like a heart pumping at the centre of a great fragrance." [38]

It is actually the aquillaria crassana tree and generally from Far East (Cambodia for example).

* * *

**It is not an amber resin as such.

BUKHUR: A preparation made from agarwood and other woods, roots, barks, and resins such as myrrh and frankincense, bound in syrup. There are hundreds of bukhur formulae, some dating back one thousand years.

Origin: originally bukhur was prepared in the high mountains of Yemen. It was sent throughout Arabia by the Queen of Yemen on auspicious occasions such as Ramadan. Bukhur is used in Islamic holy cities such as Mecca, during religious celebrations, and shared with guests as a token of great hospitality.

Although largely used in Islamic ceremonies or by Islamic people, bukhur is referred to in Christian literature and was used by the kings of England as an offering at the Feast of Epiphany.

Bukhur is found to aid concentration, improve memory, awaken the mind, enliven the spirit, and repel negative psychic forces.*

Bukhur is also haemostatic, antiseptic, anti-inflammatory, and carminative and can be applied topically to wounds.

* * *

SPIKENARD (nardostachys jatamansi, muskroot) is another herb referred to in the Old and New Testament.

Spikenard is in the same plant family as valerian.

Spikenard (not to be confused with aralia racemosa, American spikenard), was transported from the Himalayas to the Holy Land in alabaster jars. It was (and is) extremely rare and expensive. It was used by Mary (the sister of Lazarus) to anoint Christ at the Passover. Judas Iscariot (the keeper of the money bag) complained, saying the pot of ointment could be sold for a year's wages and the money given to the poor.[39]

Spikenard was also referred to by Homer[40] and listed by Pliny as one of twelve species of nard; and used cosmetically by the Empress Nur Jehan.

Spikenard was also mentioned twice in The Song of Solomon (1:12 and 4:13), and in Book 18 of Homer's Iliad.

---

*There are no double-blind trials to support these claims.

Uses: spikenard soothes the nervous system, is a cooling, sedative tranquilizer.

Spikenard is used as incense in the Himalayas, to drive away evil spirits.

N.B. Overuse can cause sluggishness.

The CITES (Convention on International Trade in Endangered Species) status of spikenard (jatamansi) is listed as vulnerable, and it is banned as an export from Nepal and Uttar Pradesh.

Dalby, A, (2000), *Dangerous Tastes: the story of spices,* London: British Museum Press. pp 83–88

www.biblefragrances.com

www.planetherbs.com/

Inspired Times: A much-abridged version of this and the previous article was published by *Inspired Times Magazine* www.inspiredtimesmagazine.com

* * *

LABDANUM: One of my earlier experiences of the power of scent came from cistus creticus (rockrose, labdanum), a plant known from ancient Greek and Egyptian legend. My wife and I had been invited to a cistus farm in Northern Crete, where we received wonderful hospitality and the opportunity to observe the collection of labdanum. Hippocrates first mentioned the combing of goats' hair to collect labdanum in the fifth century BC.

The resin-soaked goat hair was burned as incense and also worn as false beards by ancient pharaohs.[41] Even the ancient queens of Egypt and Persia wore beards made from goat hair and labdanum to give a sense of power and authority. For example, one of the world's most ancient monuments, The Sphinx, combines a winged bearded goddess with the body of a lion.

It is thought that the myrrh of the Old and New Testament was actually drawn from labdanum rather than comniphora myrrha or common myrrh. Medusa and Poseidon were thought to live in a cistus grove. The plant, first recorded in Crete, was sacred to the goddess Aphrodite.

41

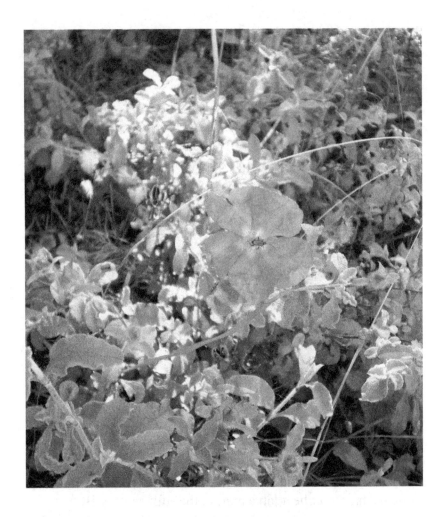

The resin from rockrose (cistus species) has a smell reminiscent of ambergris; it is antiviral, antibacterial, stimulant, expectorant, emmenagogue, anti-inflammatory, and is said to be useful in cases of bronchitis and urinary infections. In the Unani tradition, cistus is described as cold and moist in the first degree.

There are connections between rockrose and other biblical plants, such as rose of Sharon (commonly thought to be in the hypericum family) and balm of Gilead (associated with the balsam poplar from North America).

"To prevent hair loss, rub head with oil of cistus or oil of myrtle." [42] Hakim Chishti

My gratitude goes to Dimitris Nyktaris for giving me the opportunity to investigate and experience this plant.

Dimitris Nyktaris (http:chypre-perfume.blogspot.com)

CHAPTER EIGHT

Fragrances of the Season—The Florals

Consider the Lilies

I suppose this piece started when I was talking to my herb class about the attributes of lily of the valley as an attar or pure perfume essence. One of the qualities of this perfume was described by Hakim Chishti as "rekindling pleasant memories of the past." A week or two later I was asked to give a talk to the local herb society, and before introducing me, the secretary presented a short profile on snowdrops, stating that a pharmaceutical company was now using one of its active ingredients, galanthine (or galantamine), as a medicine for treating Alzheimer's. Another herbalist interjected and said that now the pharmaceutical industry is using galanthine from daffodils as it is cheaper and more plentiful than that extracted from either snowdrops (galanthus) or lily of the valley.

So here I am on a sunny afternoon, sitting in my garden surrounded by spring flowers and marvelling at the way nature always provides us with what we need when we need it most.

I'd been researching natural medicines for Alzheimer's, and apart from a great deal of research on the effect of herbs such as ginkgo biloba, gotu kola, vinca minor, and fish oils on mental acuity, I now have become alerted to the fact that the pharmaceutical industry is synthesizing galanthine from daffodils.

Galanthine is a substance present in many spring and summer flowers, including lily of the valley, daffodils, hyacinth, and snowdrops.

Snowdrops were used traditionally by Russian people to ease nerve pain, and it was this and other observations that encouraged Russian and Bulgarian scientists to do further research resulting in the active ingredient galanthine being isolated in 1958 and becoming commercially available in 1984. It is, of course, extremely expensive (another bit of pocket money for the pharmaceutical giants).

I often recommend attar (pure perfume essence) of lily of the valley for "rekindling pleasant memories of the past" and have recently acquired a small amount of attar of nargis (wild daffodil), which although having a totally different perfume, with a rich golden colour and a musky fragrance reminiscent of young amber and saffron, appears to have a similar psychological effect.

"Their sweet perfume was thought to be as dangerous as any narcotic." [43]

And now galanthamine (originally taken from the Caucasian snowdrop galanthus woronowii) is being used by the pharmaceutical companies in the treatment of mild to moderate Alzheimer's. I sincerely hope the scientists remember that it was traditional herbalists who first discovered the properties of these plants before it was deemed necessary to isolate, synthesize, and validate what was already known.

Other attars (natural perfumes) of spring and summer flowers include rose (more than a hundred different types of rose are used), Persian lilac, honeysuckle, Tunisian jasmine, French gardenia, and the Arabic blend known as Al Nabha (The Spring).

All of these have known physical and mental health benefits.

* * *

NARGIS:

Nargis (narcissi pseudonarcissus) was first mentioned in the sixth century by Mohammed and was used by mediaeval Arabs as a cure for baldness (which means that it stimulates the scalp in the same way that other brain tonics such as gotu kola and bacopa do). The word 'narcissus' comes from the Greek word for numbness, referring to the narcotic properties of the plant. Roman soldiers carried daffodil bulbs into battle in case of mortal wounding; the bulb would be eaten to ensure a painless death.

* * *

NEROLI:

In Marrakesh an herb supplier had sold my wife a bottle of neroli oil, which had leaked into her cloth toiletries bag as we travelled south to Essouira. That night in our room I placed the bag on a storage heater to dry, filling the air with the perfume of neroli. We both slept for ten hours.

On returning to Marrakesh a week or so later, we went back to the supplier and told him what had happened; not only did he replace the neroli, but it was even stronger than the one that had leaked.

Neroli was named after a town near Rome, whose sixteenth century princess wore the perfume and made it famous.

* * *

LILY OF THE VALLEY: (convallaria)

Relates to compassion, consolation, oxygen, and spring sweetness.

Lily of the valley is a plant for the heart, for all symptoms accompanying cardiac weakness. It has a digitalis-like action (only milder) and also reduces heartache (of the sentimental kind).

As an attar or natural perfume it is used to summon up pleasant memories of the past.

An ancient distillation of the flowers of lily of the valley was known as aqua aurea (golden water) and stored in vessels of gold and silver.

The sixteenth century herbalist Doedens pointed out that aqua aurea: "Doth strengthen the memorie and comforteth the Harte."

And Culpepper (seventeenth century herbalist and astrologer) stated: "It without doubt strengthens the brain and renovates a weak memory." [44]

Properties: Diuretic, emetic, purgative, heart tonic (slows heart—as with digitalis), helps promote recall of pleasant events and memories of childhood. Lily of the valley is considered a spiritually oriented fragrance.

References:

"Snowdrops: The heralds of spring and a modern drug for Alzheimer's disease." *The Pharmaceutical Journal.* Vol 273. No. 7330, p 905-906.

Heinrich M, Teoh H.L. "Galanthamine from snowdrop — the development of a modern drug against Alzheimer's disease from local Caucasian knowledge." *Journal of Ethnopharmacology,* 2004.

* * *

ROSE: "Queen of flowers" (Sappho 600 BC)

"All is permitted the rose—splendour, a conspiracy of perfumes, petalous flesh that tempts the nose, the lips, the teeth . . ." Colette

In traditional Chinese medicine, rose works on the shen aspect (heart, spirit)—but is generally considered in aromatherapy as a base note—it is cooling and grounding.

The traditional term "rose otto" comes from attar (essence or perfume in Arabic).

Rose helps with anxiety, depression, insomnia, and sudden stress. It is useful for thrush, dry skin, headaches and migraine, and has wound-healing properties. Rose can also help with hormonal issues, lifts the spirit, and drives away melancholy.

Symbolism: offers beauty, but then warns of dangers.

"Sub rosa" (to be kept in confidence) relates to the ceiling rose popular in council chambers and Christian confessionals.

Attar of roses was known by Avicenna to be cold and dry in the second degree. It is commonly used in all cases where heat is the major problem.

Roses existed thirty-five million years ago, according to fossil evidence, and were cultivated more than five thousand years ago in Asia and Africa.

Rose water became legal tender in the seventeenth century.

More than a hundred species of roses are used in medicine for their tonic, astringent, and carminative properties and are used in gargles, enemas, teas, and salves to treat everything from mouth ulcers to uterine bleeding.

Roses are rich in the bioflavonoid quercetin, vitamin C, and many other nutrients. The perfume of rose works directly on the heart and features in many of the "Soul Station" medicines.

* * *

MARIGOLD: We had arrived at the Moroccan town of Oualidia, a town fringing a lagoon, famed for its oysters. One morning as we walked along the shore of the lagoon, a local boatman offered us an hour's boat ride at a reasonable price. We circled the lagoon, coming to the opposite bank, where acres of marigolds flowered. I asked the boatman the Arabic name of these plants, and he told me *wardh*. A week later on visiting an herb supplier in Marrakesh, I asked for some *wardh*. The herbalist gave me a quizzical look before telling me "wardh means flower."

(I later found it was also a term sometimes applied to the rose but never to marigolds.) Although the marigolds in Oualidia and other parts of Morocco are calendula, it is the French or African marigold (Tagetes erecta) that is used in the preparation of marigold attar (genda). Marigolds are steam distilled in sandalwood oil to produce this interesting fragrance.

Genda: (marigold) is antimicrobial, inspires deep breathing, is useful for yoga and meditation, and is fortifying and deeply calming.

The name of the European marigold (calendula) comes from the same root as calendar. The first day of the month is associated with the sun. Its name also comes from "Mary's Gold" and is associated with the Virgin Mary. Marigolds were used to decorate church altars. Marigolds are also popular in the Hindu tradition, where they are associated with Ganesh, the mover of obstacles, and other deities.

The French or African marigold "tagetes" (which actually comes from South America) was named after Tages the grandson of Jupiter.

Marigold is often used (as is safflower) as a cheaper substitute for saffron.

* * *

JASMINE: (chameli, sien hing hwa, yasmin)
Tunisian, Egyptian, Indian (Kachu Kali), and other jasmines are uplifting while being relaxing. Jasmine is anticancer, is a calmative, antidepressant, and aphrodisiac essence, and is mainly used to calm the nervous system.

Jasmine flowers are pressed with olive oil between glass or gauze frames (the flowers are changed many times). It takes approximately thirty-one pounds of flowers to one pound of oil to produce high-quality attar.

The mystic whirling dervishes of Turkey favour jasmine.

Jasmine uplifts moods and lessens depression.

CHAPTER NINE

Base Notes—
Woody and Resinous Attars

Base notes come from various sources, including resins (such as labdanum from cistus or rockrose), lichens (oakmoss), barks (including sandalwood), grasses (such as vetivert and patchouli), and animal secretions (including musk and ambergris).

It is the base note attars that retain the perfumes' duration and hold down or anchor other essences in the attar (rose and amber, for example).

Although I may use terms such as combinations or blends, attar ingredients are distilled together rather than blended in the way essential oils might be.

SANDALWOOD:

Sandalwood cools the brain and is specific for meditation. It is a base note in aromatherapy.

Sandalwood helps with constipation, nausea, loss of appetite, anxiety, depression, insomnia, asthma, bronchitis, flu symptoms, dry eczema, sunburn, nerve pain, kidney function, and hormone balance.

FRANKINCENSE: A major attar for protection.

Frankincense can be used for all types of protection, whether physical or emotional. It lifts depression and can help with cystitis.

Frankincense is specific for enhancing memory with Alzheimer's and amnesia.

AMBER:

Amber has been described as the male counterpart to rose, will calm heart and spirit, and will work on the liver and the glandular system (including adrenals).

MUSK:

Musk can be either animal or plant origin. It is useful in the removal of negative influences and traditionally worn by Arab women following menses to balance the internal environment.

Musk is also used for fainting, dizziness, and palpitations.

Musk attar elicits raw animal energy.

OUDH: (oud, eaglewood, agarwood, aquillaria species, jin-koh, ch'en xiang)

Oudh is a resinous wood taken from ancient trees. The resin is produced as a natural immune response to parasitic growths and therefore mainly found in infected trees; as a result, oudh is becoming exceedingly rare and expensive.

Oudh is the epitome of attar and links to the highest stations of the soul; it is relaxing, tonifying, and protective.

Avicenna recommended oudh for those who suffered from depression, anxiety, palpitations, heart diseases, nausea, coughs, and body pains.

Oudh is highly cherished and traded amongst Unani, Ayurvedic, and Chinese healers; exotic oil traders, alchemists, and religious leaders; and is referred to in Biblical and other religious texts.

The resinous wood is burned on charcoal and releases a perfume that inspires a relaxed positivity. Oudh can also be purchased as attar and is often priced in the region of £500–£5,000 per ounce, depending on age, quality, and origin.

The perfume of oudh attars can vary from a rich, almost faecal smell to sweeter, spicier fragrances.

PATCHOULI: (pogostemon)

Oil extracted from the leaves and stem of the patchouli plant is known to calm the mind, acting as an antidepressant, antibacterial, antiseptic, mild aphrodisiac, memory stimulant, and being generally grounding.

"There was a young lady named Julie, who was terribly fond of Patchouli. She used bottles seven, 'til she smelt up to heaven, which made all the angels unruly." [45]

Medicinal Uses: stimulant, tonic, calmative, aphrodisiac, eases pain, useful for lung disorders (including asthma, TB). Patchouli calms and nourishes the heart.

CHAPTER TEN

Fragrance in the Time of COVID-19

"There are some things learned when we are sick and suffering that simply cannot be learned in any other way." Hakim Chishti.

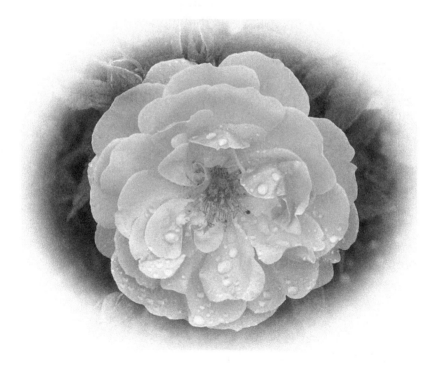

ROSE: The flower of love, magic, hope, and mystery.

"Ring a ring of roses a pocketful of posies, atishoo, atishoo we all fall down."

It is thought that the above song was written during the seventeenth century plague and that roses were not only used to cover the smell of death but also used in herbal potions by the sage Nostradamus to reduce symptoms of fever.

I am writing this during the COVID-19 pandemic, the biggest plague since the Spanish Flu (1918–1919), which killed more than fifty million people worldwide.

Today I am straining rosa damascena to add to some of my herbal blends and adding rosa creticus to my oil burner.

In traditional Chinese medicine, rose works on the shen aspect (heart, spirit)—it is generally considered in aromatherapy as a base note—it is cooling and grounding.

Rose is known to have a cooling effect on the blood, useful in treating fevers but also for calming stress and anxiety, a big issue when housebound and with friends and neighbours getting sick and dying.

"That which we call a rose by any other name would smell as sweet." [46]

Roses are not necessarily sweet. There are more than a hundred different roses used in herbal medicine and perfumery, ranging from the delicate wild roses to the darker, more sultry black roses of the Sudan and Somalia.

The traditional term "rose otto" comes from attar (essence or perfume in Arabic).

Rose promotes love and compassion, helps with anxiety, depression, insomnia, and sudden stress. It is useful for thrush, dry skin, headaches and migraine, and has wound-healing properties. Rose can also help with hormonal issues.

LAVENDER

In a time when washing our hands has become almost an obsession, perhaps it's time to take a look at lavender. In earlier plagues, lavender leaves were rubbed into the hands frequently and even worn in face masks by the plague doctors. The word lavender comes from the Latin "lavare" (to wash).

It takes around 1,000 kilos of lavender to make five kilos of distilled lavender essence, but a pot of strong lavender decoction makes an excellent hair rinse.

Lavender also "helps the panting and passion of the heart." [47]

JASMINE

This is my attar of choice for supporting the emotions. In terms of Ayurveda, jasmine is thought to balance the three doshas (body types) and support harmony in the five elements.

This attar is "unparalleled in its ability to lessen depression" [48] and has been hailed by German scientists to be as powerfully effective as Valium. [49]

JUNIPER (juniperus communis)

Often in herbal medicine, the answer is in the name. In Tibet, high-mountain juniper is used to treat community disorders such as epidemics. We also find a similar use for juniper in alchemical spagyric medicine, where key words relating to this herb include community, mass, epidemic, and contagion. Some years ago, when visiting the Grand Canyon in Arizona, I gathered some high-mountain juniper berries (pinus cedrus). Later that day we visited a Navajo trading post. My wife (a keen jeweller) was talking to the Navajo regarding their colourful beads, while I (as an herbalist) was checking out the medicine pouches. One of the pouches seemed to contain beads, so, not wanting to open the pouch, I took it to the desk and asked what was inside. The man emptied the pouch onto the desk and told me they were juniper berries. I took my berries out of my pocket and said, "But these are juniper berries. They don't look anything like yours."

"Ah, yes," he replied, "but you gathered yours from a tree. Mine were gathered from the ground, after the ants had found them and eaten the skin before boring into the berry to get at the nectar inside." (This was why his berries looked like beads ready to thread.)

So I asked the man, "What do you use them for?"

"We use them to protect the tribe," he responded. (The Navajo also use juniper to flavour tobacco.) So Tibet, Western alchemy, and the Navajo Nation all use juniper for the same thing, although these traditions are far apart.

In Morocco juniper heartwood (cade) is also used to treat psoriasis conditions (taken from juniperus oxycedrus).

A particular species of juniper (juniperus phoenicea) grows on Mount Sinai.

Herodotus referred to a substance described as "kedros" (sef wan), which appears to have been oil of juniper.

Juniper was often used in the ancient Egyptian perfume "kyphi" along with saffron and spikenard.

As an herb, juniper is useful in the treatment of bladder infections, being antiseptic, antimicrobial, antioxidant, diuretic, and anti-inflammatory.

It was also recommended to massage the body with juniper oil before an expected fever attack.

"Juniper strengthens the brain and nerves."[50]

Juniper keywords include epidemic, contagion, fear, hope, protection, and purification. [51]

Afsharzadeh M., Naderinasab M., Tayarani Najaran Z., Barzin M., Emami S. A. In vitro antimicrobial activities of some Iranian conifers. *Iran J Pharm Res*. 2013; 12(1):63-74.24250573.

Carpenter C. D., O'Neill T., Picot N., et al. Anti-mycobacterial natural products from the Canadian medicinal plant *Juniperus communis*. *J Ethnopharmacol*. 2012, 143(2):695-700.22877928.

Cavaleiro C., Pinto E., Gonçalves M. J., Salgueiro L. Antifungal activity of *Juniperus* essential oils against dermatophyte, *Aspergillus* and *Candida* strains. *J Appl Microbiol*. 2006, 100(6):1333-1338.16696681.

CHAPTER ELEVEN

The Exotics

A ll attars and fragrances are exotic in their own way, so this term may be a little erroneous and could easily include rose, lotus, etc., but I did want to separate those below from the categories used so far.

TUBEROSE: (sugadaraja) "King of fragrances" "Mistress of the Night"—India. *Wan xiang yu* "flowers precious as jade and becoming fragrant at night," (China).
Tuberose is a relaxing sedative.

OSMANTHUS: a fragrance useful in decreasing irritation, stress, depression, and apathy.

ORCHID: Vanilla orchid was thought to promote strength in the Aztec culture. The orchid was favoured by Confucius in ancient China.

KEWDA: (kewra, screwpine, pandanas odorifer). Kewda is used to heal degenerative disorders. It has anti-inflammatory properties, has been used in nasal drops to treat convulsions due to epilepsy, and has blood tonifying, circulatory, and nervine properties. Only the male flowers are used for perfume, just distilling 3 to 5 percent of the oil with sandalwood.

KADAM: (kadamba, anthocephalus cadamba). Kadam fragrance is extracted from the flowers that blossom between three and six a.m. during the monsoon season. Kadam is the symbol of the infinite potential of love and wisdom. Its fragrance helps to unfold love in the heart. Kadam has analgesic and antiseptic properties, can relieve stress and depression, and is good for treating disorders of the spleen (which may give rise to worry and pensiveness).

MAJMUA: containing ruh khus (heart of vetivert), mitti (sweet earth), and kadam (Indonesian flowering tree associated with good fortune).

AMBERGRIS: So there I was in 1972, strolling along a stretch of Bombay Beach and stepping on something brownish and smelly. On removing it from my shoe, I realized that it wasn't what I assumed it to be and had an interesting smell and texture. I wrapped the substance in an old copy of *The Times of India* and took it to a friendly Ayurvedic medicine supplier in the back streets. "Hah," he said, nodding his head from side to side. "This is ambergris, and it is worth one thousand rupees." (I don't remember the price he quoted and paid me after a lengthy discussion, but I know that it bought me a good lunch, paid my fare to Kashmir, and got me a room on Dhal Lake.)

I tend to describe ambergris as "whale vomit"; it is created in the intestines of the sperm whale by excess irritants, including squid beaks, and ejected rather like a cat ejects an offending furball (but not necessarily from the same orifice).

Ambergris contains *ambrein,* used by perfumers to extend the duration of a fragrance.

Ambergris was known in early Arab civilizations as *"anbar"* and used in the treatment of the brain, heart, and sense organs.

"When Anbar is inhaled, it relieves flu symptoms, headaches, and migraine." [52]

"Ambergris—do you know where it comes from? It's coughed up by the sperm whale when it devours cuttlefish. It's a greenish, revolting mass that floats on the surface of the ocean, ripening in the sun and rain until it's washed ashore. And yet from these humble beginnings develops the most indescribable scent, it literally expands on the skin—creates a vista in the senses." [53]

AMBER: (unbar, ambergris) "King of Scents."

As a gemstone, amber is considered capable of preserving or restoring strength and vitality. In some countries it is worn by brides to ensure happiness and long life and by warriors for protection in battle. In China, amber is called The Soul of the Tiger and worn as a symbol of courage. In Tibet, amber is an emblem of good fortune, health, and success. Amber axes were placed in ancient Scandinavian tombs as a symbol of immortality.

Amber is either taken from the whale (ambergris—as above) or taken from a tree resin (cypress family). It is generally considered to be the masculine counterpart to the rose. Amber promotes balance and relaxation and relates to mystery and ancient ritual.

Amber works on the endocrine system and is therefore good for the chronically ill. Not best at night, as it may stimulate.

MUSK: can be either of animal or plant origin (deer, civet, or ambrette seed from the hibiscus).

Deer musk is only produced by the male deer and is used to mark its territory and attract females.

"Art thou musk or ambergris, for I am charmed by thy delicious smell."[54]

Musk is useful in removing negative influences and in repelling psychic imbalances. It's traditionally worn by Arab women following menses to balance the internal environment. This perfume creates an aura of excellence and purity while eliciting raw animal energy.

In Islam, musk was mixed into the mortar of early mosques.

Musk can also be used to treat fainting, dizziness, and palpitations.

MITTI: Baked Earth. "The smell of rain."

"Exhalation of moss, mycelium, black mould; wafted savor of a thousand earthy growths, damp, clinging, redolent; aroma of mighty roots, of invisible spawn and seed—all the vast stirring. Earth and rain, dust and desire, what mingled odour of these is not sweet?"[55]

As streams flow down the mountains from the Himalayan snows, they pass through flower meadows, where Tibetan pony traders gather to rest.

Streams then descend into the fern-clad woodlands, forming greater rivers, before entering the pine forests, continuing to Gaumukh to form the Ganges.

The Ganges then flows through birch trees, whose bark was used to write the first Vedic texts.

On the way, river mud becomes impregnated with the perfume of the plants the river encounters.

When the first monsoons arrive, releasing the smell of the first rain, portions of the Ganges mud are hydro-distilled with sandalwood oil, creating a most exotic attar.

Similar results are produced in other great and sacred rivers, including the Nile.

Mitti has a calming, cooling, and grounding quality.

SHAFAYAT: The Healer

I will never forget one of my earlier talks on attars, which I gave to a group of practitioners from various herbal traditions. I was halfway through my talk when I became aware that sitting in a dark corner of the room was a hakim from the Unani tradition who probably knew more about attars than I will ever know. I continued my talk with a certain trepidation. When I had finished and answered several questions, the hakim approached me and said, "That was an excellent talk, but just one thing: you mispronounced Shafayat—it should be 'Shafaya'at.'" I met the hakim many times over the years that followed and even bought attars from him, which had been delivered from Saudi Arabia in a diplomatic bag.

Shafaya'at contains at least six attars, including amber, sandalwood, and frankincense. The Healer enlivens the mind, produces positive thoughts, and creates a mood of balanced confidence.

HAJR E ASWAD: The Black Stone

"The Black Stone descended from Paradise, and it was whiter than milk, then it was blackened by the sins of the children of Adam."[56]

The black stone of Mecca was said to have descended from heaven. It is covered by a black silk cloth (kiswa), which is embroidered with silver and gold.

The covering of the stone is perfumed and purified before prayers with a combination of attars, including oudh and sandalwood.

BLUE NILE: Rumoured to be the perfume worn by Cleopatra and based upon the flowers and barks that the queen used in her bath, including jasmine and lotus, but minus the ass's milk. Blue Nile is an exotic and uplifting attar, known for lightening the mood.

JANNAT AL FERDOUS: "Gateway to the Highest Paradise." The story regarding this attar comes from the experience of a whirling dervish who ascended into the clouds. When questioned on his return as to where he'd been, he said, "I have been to heaven and intend to emulate the perfume I smelled there."

The word Jannat is Turkish for heaven (Jannah in Arabic). Firdous refers to the highest garden of heaven.

Jannat al Ferdous will generally contain jasmine (favoured by dervishes) lotus, gardenia, sandalwood, musk, and other fragrances.

CHAPTER TWELVE

Pure Perfumes (Attars) to Enhance Presence, Confidence, and Well-Being

Single Attars

FRANKINCENSE & MYRRH—Protection, purification, spirituality.

FRANGIPANI—Hospitality, love.

HENNA—*"The Lord of sweet-smelling blossoms in this world and the next."* [57] Strengthens mind and body, rejuvenates, alterative, nervine tonic, tranquilizer, enhances circulation.

HINA—(henna) Recommended by Mohammed for pain in the legs.

HONEYSUCKLE—Money, psychic power.

LILAC—Protection (early morning).

LILY—Protection, grief.

LILY OF THE VALLEY—Happiness, mental powers. Lily of the valley not only awakens the heart but also brings memories of pleasant events.

MITTI—"the scent of the first rains" Calming, cooling, grounding.

MUSK—Attraction, lust. Used to purify and protect, especially during vulnerable times.

PATCHOULI—Calms the mind, antidepressant, antibacterial, antiseptic, mild aphrodisiac, memory stimulant, grounding.

ROSE—(cooling) Romantic, aphrodisiac, mild laxative, antidepressant, promotes immunity.

SAFFRON—(warming) Blood cleanser, improves colour of complexion, enhances clarity of perception, decongestant, aphrodisiac, balances hormones.

NARCISSUS—Love, fertility, luck.

PERSIAN LILAC—Reminiscent of a spring morning.

Rose, jasmine, and saffron are used to calm the spirit of the heart, whereas amber and other woody extracts work on heart, liver, and endocrine systems.

The more sultry tones of certain ambers, musk, oudh, and night rose have quite sensual fragrances.

The above represents just a handful of the hundreds of fragrances used in this system of medicine. Attars can be used therapeutically, intuitively, or sensually—their range of application is without bounds.

Specific combinations:

Bedroom Blend: amber, rose and musk (applied to nape of neck and wrists).

(Erogenous attars include costus and musk—sultry notes will include jasmine, styrax, labdanum, and tuberose).

General Fatigue: Amber, musk (use in bath or massage of the nape of the neck).

Lack of Life Force: Sandalwood, frankincense (in bath or nape of neck).

Oversensitivity: Sandalwood, frankincense (in an oil burner or as perfume).

Pure Emotion: Rose, lily of the valley (apply to nape of neck and wrists).

To enhance personal power: Frankincense, amber, and violet (fragrance on wrist points, in right ear ridge with cotton, or on shoulder blades).

To gain self-confidence: Amber, frankincense, myrrh, and violet (as fragrance—nape of neck, right ear ridge with cotton).

To gain greater respect from others: Frankincense, myrrh, violet, musk, and patchouli (nape of neck, ridge of right ear with cotton).

To increase concentration: Myrrh, frankincense, patchouli (oil burner or as perfume).

To heal wounds of the heart: Myrrh (in the bath or as perfume).

To improve or sharpen memory: Sandalwood, frankincense (in an oil burner or as perfume).

To reduce depression: Jasmine, lily of the valley (as perfume or in oil burner).

To purify the environment: Frankincense, patchouli (in an oil burner).

To promote sleep: Violet (in the bath or as fragrance, nape of neck, soles of feet).

PMS, feeling overheated: Amber, rose, musk (in the bath or as fragrance).

Selfishness, arrogance, and/or self-deception: Violet, rose, sandalwood (oil burner or perfume).

Rose, jasmine, and bergamot blend with almost everything.

Attars might be worn due to perfume preference or personal physical or emotional need. They can also be used to strengthen specific organ functions.

Brain: responds well to musk, jasmine, oudh, and frankincense.

Heart: to Sandalwood, rose, amber, oudh, and hyacinth.

Liver: Amber.

Stomach: Rose, oudh.

Female Reproductive System: Olive (in the Attari tradition, "aged" olive oil is used), rose, sandalwood.

Male Reproductive System: Myrrh, musk, lily of the valley, violet, amber.

* * *

Attars, as with plants, will be influenced by the planets or have a "ruling planet."

Ruling Planets:

Aries's ruler: Mars, which responds well to myrrh and spikenard.

Taurus's rulers: Venus, responds well to sandalwood, myrrh, and rose.

Gemini's ruler: Mercury, responds well to lavender.

Cancer's ruler: Moon, jasmine, ylang ylang.

Leo's ruler: Sun, frankincense, and myrrh.

Virgo's rulers: Mercury, lavender.

Libra's ruler: Venus, responds well to sandalwood, myrrh, and rose.

Scorpio's rulers: Mars (ancient) and Pluto (modern).

Sagittarius's ruler: Jupiter.

Capricorn's ruler: Saturn.

Aquarius's rulers: Saturn (ancient) and Uranus (modern).

Pisces's rulers: Jupiter (ancient) and Neptune (modern).

Some examples:

Frankincense: protection, spirituality; ruler: sun; star sign: Leo.

Jasmine: calming yet uplifting; ruler: moon; star sign: Cancer

Kewda: (pandanus—screw pine) converting stress to positivity; ruler: Mars; star signs: Aries, Scorpio.

Rose: all matters relating to the heart; ruler: Venus; star signs: Taurus, Libra.

Sandalwood: tranquillity, meditation, (applied to the brow chakra); ruler: Venus + Jupiter; star signs: Taurus, Libra, Sagittarius.

Regardless of ancestry, tradition, physical, mental, emotional, spiritual condition, star sign, or planetary configuration, attars can be used simply because they smell good!

Acknowledgements

Much of this chapter has been taken from the writings of Hakim Chishti.

The Canon of Medicine: (al Qanun fi'l—tibb) Avicenna— Adapted by Laleh Bakhtiar.

Unani: The Science of Graeco-Arabic Medicine. Prof. Jamil Ahmad, Hakim Ashtar Qadeer. Lustre Press 1998.

Schrott et al *Marma Therapy* 2016.

REFERENCES

(Others are cited in chapters above)

A Modern Herbal, Grieve, Mrs. M., Reprinted by Penguin Books—1980.

Aromatica, A Clinical Guide to Essential Oil Therapeutics; Volume 1 Principles and Profiles. 2016. + Volume 2. Applications and Profiles. 2019. Holmes P. Singing Dragon, London and Philadelphia.

An Ancient Egyptian Herbal, Lise Manniche. The American University in Cairo Press. 2006.

"Avicenna—The Prince of Physicians." H.M. Chishti. *East West—The Journal of Natural Health & Living.* August 1986.

David Crowe L.Ac (Floracopeia)

Dimitris Nyktaris (http:chypre-perfume.blogspot.com)

"Essence & Alchemy" Mandy Aftel. Bloomsbury 2001.

Ibn Sina and Farid al Din Attar: Two Versions of the Legend of the Wandering Bird Souls to God. Julia E. Fedorova, PhD. Research Fellow, Department of Philosophy of the Islam Institute of Philosophy, Russia.

The Canon of Medicine: (al Qanun fi'l—tibb) Avicenna—Adapted by Laleh Bakhtiar.

Marma Therapy Schrott et al 2016, Singing Dragon.

The Occult Properties of Herbs—W. B. Crow. The Aquarian Press, 1969.

BBC News, 2009.

Qazi Shaikh Abbas Borhany, Qasi Habibullah.

Syedi Abdulqadir bin Qazi Habibullah, *"Al Risalatil Nadira Fil Attur al Fakhirah"* manuscript, Hiraz, Yemen.

The Oman Observer

Unani: The Science of Graeco-Arabic Medicine. Prof. Jamil Ahmad, Hakim Ashtar Qadeer. Lustre Press 1998.

Willard, P. (2001) *Secrets of Saffron: The Vagabond Life of the World's Most Seductive Spice,* Beacon Press. Retrieved 2009.

Yemen Times, Issue 863, Volume 13.

END NOTES

1   Michael Edwards from *Fragrances of the World.*

2   *Perfume* by Patrick Suskind,—p 200—Penguin Fiction, 1987.

3   'On cold effleurage'—from *Perfume* by Patrick Suskind—p 186.

4   Importance of Sense of Smell, by Helen Keller.

5   Genesis 2.7

6   Thoth is often depicted with the head of an ibis, to represent the pen or quill. He was considered to be the inventor of hieroglyphics and thought by some historians to be the author of *The Egyptian Book of the Dead.* Thoth is also thought to be synonymous with Hermes—the founder of alchemy and a contemporary of Moses.

7   Tabitha Morgan, BBC News, Nicosia.

8   This particular snake is referred to as *Tyr* and believed to be the painted saw-scaled viper (*echis colorata*) found in the Sinai region.

9   Ramban commentary to Exodus 30–34.

10   Lord Krishna—*Bhagavad Gita* v11.9

11   Lad V—Marma Points in Ayurveda

12   Farooq 1998

13   Lise Manniche (An Ancient Egyptian Herbal)

14   Alice Poon, "Orchids and Confucius," *Asia Sentinel*, 2008.

15   Exodus 30.

16   *African Journal of Biochemistry Research* Vol. 5(7), pp. 214–219, July 2011

17   *Shen Nong Ben Cao (Divine Husbandman's Classic of the Materia Medica).*

18   Ikeda, T et al. Cytotoxic Glycosides form Albizzia julibrissin, J. Nat. Prod. 1997, 60, 102-107.

19   Exodus 30–34/35 (King James Version)

20   Psalms 45:8

21   Song of Songs 4: 13-14

22   Solomon 4:14

23   Apocryphal Book of Enoch

24   Mahmoud Suhail (immunologist)

25   "Guggulipid for the treatment of hypercholesterolemia: a randomised control trial." *JAMA*, August 13, 2003 290(6): 765–72, Szapary, P.O., et al.

26 Sufi Farid al Din Attar (1145–1221 approx.) wrote "The Conference of the Birds" (Mantiq al-Tayr); Ibn Sina (980–1037) wrote "The Message of the Birds (Risulat al-Tayr), which was translated from Arabic to Farsi in 1191. It was Ibn Sina who first used birds as a metaphor for the soul. Ibn Sina was also the first to distill roses (rose attar). Sufi Attar was known as "The Perfumer" and was said to have written "The Conference of the Birds" in his pharmacy from where he prescribed medicines and perfumes.

27 Aristotle claimed that the heart was the first organ to be developed in the fetus; Hippocrates claimed it was the brain. It is interesting to note that ancient Chinese illustrations of the source of shen (heart/mind/spirit—the phoenix) combines both.

28 Each nasal passage has a small (2.5 cm square) area containing fifty million sensory receptor cells, which send messages to the olfactory bulb (a projection of the brain). From the olfactory bulb a signal is transmitted to the limbic system where memory is used to recognise odours.

 Memory can be enhanced by certain smells, such as wild daffodil (narcissus) Lily of the Valley, and Frankincense, and can be used in cases of Alzheimer's and amnesia.

 The limbic system also regulates mood and emotion. Pure plant oils (attars) can be used to release creativity, resolve disturbed emotions, and enhance beauty: rose, jasmine, amber, oudh, etc.

29 Avicenna. *The Canon of Medicine*, p 448.

30 Avicenna. *The Canon of Medicine*, p 495.

31 Fung, K., Suhail, M., & McClendon, B., Woolley, C., Young,D.G., Lin H.K. (2013). Management of basal cell carcinoma of the skin using frankincense (Boswellia sacra) essential oil: a case report. Researchgate.net, 1(2), 1–5.

 Ni, X., Suhail, M., Yang, Q., Cao, A., Fung, K.M., Postier, R.G.,Woolley, C., Young, G., Zhang, J., Lin H.K. (2012). Frankincense essential oil prepared from hydrodistillation of Boswellia sacra gum resins induces human pancreatic cancer cell death in cultures and in a. BMC Complementary andAlternative Medicine, 12, 253.

32 The Prophet Mohammed

33 The Koran

34 Sergeeva et al 2010

35 The Prophet Mohammed.

36 "Dioscorides Materia Medica"

37 Roger Bacon (thirteenth century friar and alchemist).

38 Tessaro, Kathleen. *"The Perfume Collector"*. Harper Collins 2013.

39 The New Testament: John 12:1-10.

40   Iliad
41   Dimitris Niktaris: "If you examine pictures of pharaohs or Osiris (the imagery is largely interchangeable) you will see that the arms are crossed over the chest, one hand bearing a crook (a legacy of the goat herding days), the other hand bearing a flail (ladanesterion). The pharaoh wears a false beard (even if female!) actually made from goat hair, which was evidentially stuck to the chin using labdanum."
42   Hakim Chishti
43   Wells Diana—*100 Flowers and How They Got Their Names*, 1997.
44   Culpepper—"Complete Herbal" Wordsworth Reference, 1995.
45   Ethel Watts Mumford
46   W. Shakespeare, *Romeo and Juliet,* Act 2. Scene 2.
47   John Gerard (Herbalist)
48   Hakim Chishti
49   Sergeeva et al, 2010
50   Culpepper
51   Dr J Naidu—Phylak Sachsen, 2018.
52   The Medicinal uses of Attar: from the Yemeni Treatise—By: Qazi Dr. Shaikh Abbas Borhany.
53   *The Perfume Collector*, Kathleen Tessaro, Harper Collins. 2013.
54   Saadi—thirteenth century Persian poet.
55   *Out West Magazine*, Volume 28.
56   Tirimidhi 877, Book 9: Hadith 70.
57   Farooq 1998.

CPSIA information can be obtained
at www.ICGtesting.com
Printed in the USA
LVHW082110040323
740953LV00008B/225

9 781682 352830